STRETCHING EXERCISES FOR SENIORS OVER 50

Unlock Your True Strength: The Essential Guide to Stretching for Seniors to enhance flexibility.

Desmond O. Allen

Table of Contents

Chapter 1

Introduction

Stretching is a timeless practice that transcends generations, offering a path to improved health and vitality. In the journey of aging, maintaining flexibility becomes a key aspect of overall well-being for seniors over 50. This chapter delves into the foundational principles of stretching for seniors, exploring the profound benefits it brings and the importance of tailoring exercises to suit the unique needs of this demographic.

Embracing the Benefits of Stretching

As the pages of time turn, one constant remains—the inherent benefits of stretching. In the realm of senior fitness, where the body undergoes natural changes, stretching emerges as a powerful tool to counteract the effects of aging. It's not merely about reaching for toes or performing intricate poses; it's about unlocking the body's true potential.

Stretching contributes significantly to maintaining and enhancing flexibility. Flexibility, in turn, plays a pivotal role in daily activities, from bending to tie shoelaces to reaching for items on higher shelves. Beyond the physical realm, stretching has profound effects on mental well-being. It promotes relaxation, reduces stress, and fosters a sense of calm—a valuable respite in the bustling world of today.

Moreover, embracing the benefits of stretching is not confined to the immediate moments during exercise. It ripples through time, bestowing long-term advantages. Consistent stretching helps alleviate joint stiffness, enhancing the range of motion and preserving the fluidity of movements. This is particularly crucial for seniors, as it aids in maintaining independence and an active lifestyle.

Tailoring Exercises for Seniors

One size does not fit all, especially when it comes to stretching exercises for seniors over 50. Recognizing and respecting the individuality of each person is fundamental to crafting an effective and safe stretching routine. Tailoring exercises ensures that seniors can reap the benefits without undue strain or risk.

The aging process manifests uniquely in each individual, influencing factors such as flexibility, muscle tone, and overall mobility. Therefore, a one-size-fits-all approach falls short in addressing the diverse needs of seniors. Instead, tailoring exercises involves a thoughtful consideration of personal health, fitness levels, and any existing conditions.

This tailoring process extends beyond physical aspects to encompass psychological and emotional well-being. For some, stretching may be an opportunity for gentle introspection and mindful movement. For others, it might be a social activity, fostering connections with fellow seniors in a group setting. Understanding these nuances allows for the creation of personalized stretching programs that resonate with the individual.

Moreover, tailoring exercises for seniors involves adaptability. Recognizing that mobility levels may vary, the exercises should be scalable and modifiable. A well-constructed stretching routine accommodates those who may prefer chair-based exercises due to limited mobility while providing challenges for those who can engage in standing or floor-based stretches.

In this journey of tailoring exercises, communication becomes a vital tool. Seniors are encouraged to share their experiences, preferences, and any concerns. This collaborative approach ensures that the stretching regimen aligns with individual goals and addresses specific areas of focus, whether it be improving flexibility, reducing stiffness, or simply enjoying the rejuvenating aspects of stretching.

In essence, this chapter sets the stage for a profound exploration into the world of stretching for seniors. It invites them to embrace the myriad benefits waiting to unfold and highlights the importance of customizing their stretching journey. As we embark on this odyssey, the chapters that follow will delve deeper into the principles, techniques, and routines that form the backbone of unlocking true strength through stretching.

Chapter 2

Understanding Senior Fitness

The journey into the realm of senior fitness is akin to navigating uncharted waters. As individuals gracefully traverse the sands of time, their bodies undergo a series of transformations that demand a nuanced approach to health and well-being. Chapter 2 aims to shed light on the intricacies of senior fitness, with a specific focus on the changes in flexibility that accompany the aging process and the pivotal role stretching plays in promoting vitality and resilience.

Aging Gracefully: Changes in Flexibility

Aging, a natural and inevitable part of life, bestows wisdom, experiences, and, yes, a set of physical changes. One of the key areas affected is flexibility. Understanding how flexibility evolves over time is essential for tailoring effective stretching exercises for seniors over 50.

In the early stages of life, flexibility often seems boundless. Children effortlessly bend, twist, and contort their bodies in a display of youthful suppleness. However, as the years unfold, the body undergoes a gradual metamorphosis. Collagen, the protein responsible for skin elasticity and joint health, diminishes with age. This reduction in collagen affects the connective tissues, making them less pliable and more prone to stiffness.

Joint lubrication, provided by synovial fluid, also experiences changes. With age, the production of synovial fluid decreases, leading to joints that may not move as smoothly as before. The cumulative effect of these changes is a gradual decline in the range of motion and flexibility. Simple tasks, such as reaching for objects or tying shoelaces, may become more challenging.

Muscles, too, play a pivotal role in flexibility. Over time, muscle mass tends to decrease, and the remaining fibers may become stiffer. This can affect the ability to stretch comfortably and move joints through their full range of motion. The combination of these factors underscores the need for targeted interventions to maintain and enhance flexibility in seniors.

Importance of Stretching for Seniors

In the tapestry of senior fitness, stretching emerges as a beacon of hope and resilience. Its importance extends far beyond the realm of flexibility, encompassing physical, mental, and emotional well-being. As we unravel the layers, the significance of incorporating stretching into the daily lives of seniors becomes increasingly evident.

Physical Well-being

At its core, stretching is a dynamic activity that engages muscles, joints, and connective tissues. For seniors, this engagement holds profound physical benefits. Regular stretching helps counteract the stiffness that may creep into joints, fostering a greater range of motion. Improved flexibility contributes to better posture, reducing the risk of falls and enhancing overall mobility.

Stretching also plays a pivotal role in maintaining muscle tone. As muscle mass naturally decreases with age, incorporating stretching exercises helps preserve the remaining muscle fibers. This, in turn, supports balance and stability, critical components in preventing accidents and maintaining independence.

Mental Well-being

Beyond its physical attributes, stretching exercises wield a transformative influence on mental well-being. The rhythmic, intentional movements inherent in stretching promote a sense of mindfulness and relaxation. In a world bustling with constant stimuli, the meditative qualities of stretching offer a valuable sanctuary for seniors to unwind and destress.

Moreover, the mind-body connection established through stretching fosters a heightened awareness of one's own body. Seniors become attuned to the subtle nuances of movement and sensation, creating a profound connection that transcends the physical realm. This mindfulness can extend to other aspects of life, influencing decision-making, stress management, and overall mental resilience.

Emotional Well-being

Emotions, often intertwined with physical sensations, find expression in the realm of stretching. Seniors may discover a sense of accomplishment as they gradually improve their flexibility. The release of endorphins, the body's natural feel-good chemicals, during stretching contributes to an uplifted mood.

In a societal context where social connections are vital, group stretching activities provide opportunities for camaraderie and shared experiences. Seniors coming together for stretching sessions not only reap physical benefits but also cultivate a sense of community and support. This communal aspect enhances emotional well-being, offering a platform for shared goals and mutual encouragement.

Weaving the Threads Together

As we unravel the tapestry of understanding senior fitness, the threads of aging gracefully and the importance of stretching weave together seamlessly. The changes in flexibility that accompany aging become not just markers of time but invitations to explore new avenues of self-care and resilience.

The journey into senior fitness is not a solitary one; it's a collective exploration of the body's potential and a celebration of the wisdom that comes with age. In the chapters that follow, we will delve deeper into the practical aspects of stretching exercises, providing a roadmap for seniors to unlock their true strength and embrace a life of enhanced flexibility, vitality, and well-being.

Chapter 3

Getting Started Safely

Embarking on a journey towards enhanced flexibility and well-being requires a thoughtful and deliberate approach. Chapter 3, "Getting Started Safely," lays the foundation for a safe and effective stretching routine tailored specifically for seniors over 50. Delving into the nuances of preparation and warm-up techniques, this chapter serves as a crucial guide to ensure that the path to unlocking true strength begins with careful consideration and attention to the body's needs.

Preparing for Stretching

Before delving into the invigorating world of stretching exercises, it's essential to lay a solid groundwork through thoughtful preparation. The body, much like any instrument, requires tuning and preparation to perform optimally. In the context of senior fitness, this preparatory phase becomes even more critical.

Physical Assessment

The starting point for any stretching routine is a thorough physical assessment. Understanding one's current level of flexibility, any existing physical limitations, and areas of potential concern forms the cornerstone of an effective and safe stretching program. This assessment need not be complex; it can involve simple movements to gauge the range of motion in major joints and identify any areas of stiffness or discomfort.

Seniors are encouraged to approach this assessment with curiosity and self-compassion. It is not about meeting a predefined benchmark but rather about gaining insights into the unique characteristics of one's body. This knowledge becomes the compass guiding the subsequent stretching journey, allowing for the customization of exercises to address specific needs and goals.

Health Considerations

Equally important in the preparation phase is a consideration of overall health. Seniors are advised to consult with healthcare professionals before embarking on a new fitness regimen, especially if they have pre-existing medical conditions or concerns. This consultation serves as a proactive measure to ensure that the chosen stretching exercises align with individual health goals and do not pose any risks.

For those with chronic conditions such as arthritis or osteoporosis, modifications and specific recommendations from healthcare providers can enhance the safety and efficacy of the stretching routine. By fostering an open line of communication with healthcare professionals, seniors empower themselves with the knowledge needed to make informed decisions about their fitness journey.

Setting Realistic Goals

Setting realistic and achievable goals is a pivotal aspect of preparing for stretching exercises. Rather than aiming for drastic transformations overnight, seniors are encouraged to embrace a gradual and sustainable approach. Realistic goals might include improving flexibility in a specific joint, alleviating stiffness in the lower back, or enhancing overall mobility.

These goals serve as beacons, guiding the stretching routine and providing a sense of accomplishment as milestones are achieved. Furthermore, realistic goals contribute to the establishment of a positive mindset, fostering motivation and consistency in the journey towards unlocking true strength.

Warm-up Techniques

As the saying goes, "Preparation is the key to success." This holds especially true for stretching exercises, where a well-executed warm-up sets the stage for a safe and effective session. Warm-up techniques are the gentle invitations extended to muscles and joints, inviting them to participate actively in the forthcoming stretching routine.

Cardiovascular Warm-up

Commencing the warm-up with light cardiovascular activities is akin to opening the curtains to let in the morning light. It signals the body that it's time to transition from a state of rest to one of movement. For seniors, low-impact activities such as brisk walking, stationary cycling, or gentle aerobics serve as ideal cardiovascular warm-ups.

The duration of this phase may vary based on individual fitness levels, but a general guideline is to aim for approximately 5 to 10 minutes. This gradual escalation in intensity prepares the cardiovascular system by increasing heart rate and circulation, priming the body for the stretching exercises that follow.

Dynamic Stretching

Dynamic stretching introduces controlled, fluid movements that mimic the actions expected during the stretching routine. Unlike static stretching, where positions are held for an extended duration, dynamic stretching involves continuous, rhythmic motions that progressively increase the range of motion and flexibility.

For seniors, dynamic stretches may include leg swings, arm circles, or gentle torso twists. These movements are designed to engage major muscle groups and joints, enhancing blood flow and promoting synovial fluid lubrication. Dynamic stretching not only readies the body for more intense stretching but also improves muscle coordination and responsiveness.

Joint Mobilization

Incorporating joint mobilization exercises into the warm-up further enhances the preparatory phase. These exercises focus on gently moving the joints through their natural range of motion, promoting synovial fluid distribution and reducing stiffness.

Seniors can engage in activities such as wrist circles, ankle rotations, or shoulder rolls. These exercises are particularly beneficial for individuals with arthritis or joint-related concerns, as they help improve joint flexibility and reduce discomfort associated with stiffness.

Mindful Breathing

As the warm-up progresses, integrating mindful breathing techniques becomes a valuable practice. Mindful breathing serves a dual purpose: it promotes relaxation and focuses attention on the present moment. Seniors are encouraged to engage in deep, diaphragmatic breathing during the warm-up, inhaling slowly through the nose and exhaling through pursed lips.

This intentional focus on breath not only oxygenates the body but also establishes a mind-body connection. It prepares seniors for the stretching exercises by cultivating a sense of calm and mindfulness, ensuring that the stretching routine becomes a holistic experience that transcends the physical realm.

A Holistic Approach to Getting Started

In the intricate dance of preparation and warm-up, seniors find the key to unlocking true strength. By embracing the importance of thorough preparation, conducting physical assessments, considering health factors, and setting realistic goals, individuals lay a solid foundation for their stretching journey.

Warm-up techniques become the gentle overture, inviting the body to participate willingly and actively. Cardiovascular warm-ups, dynamic stretching, joint mobilization, and mindful breathing collectively contribute to a holistic approach that not only enhances physical readiness but also fosters a sense of mindfulness and connection.

As we delve deeper into the subsequent chapters, armed with the knowledge gained in this preparatory phase, seniors are poised to embark on stretching exercises that are not just routines but transformative experiences. The path to enhanced flexibility and well-being unfolds, and each step is taken with the assurance of safety, mindfulness, and a profound understanding of the body's capabilities.

Chapter 4

Key Stretching Principles

Stretching, often viewed as a simple act of elongating muscles, transcends its apparent simplicity when approached with an understanding of key principles. In Chapter 4, "Key Stretching Principles," we delve into the fundamental aspects that form the backbone of an effective stretching routine for seniors over 50. With a focus on embracing a comprehensive approach to range of motion and harnessing the power of intentional breathing, this chapter illuminates the intricacies of unlocking true strength through mindful stretching.

Range of Motion: A Comprehensive Approach

Imagine the body as a symphony, each joint and muscle playing a unique note. The comprehensive approach to range of motion is akin to conducting this symphony, ensuring that every component moves harmoniously. In the realm of senior fitness, understanding and fostering a comprehensive range of motion is central to the success of stretching exercises.

Joint-Specific Stretching

To comprehend the comprehensive approach to range of motion, it's vital to acknowledge that different joints have unique characteristics and movement patterns.

Tailoring stretching exercises to address each joint's specific needs ensures that the entire body experiences a well-rounded and balanced range of motion.

For example, shoulders, with their intricate structure, benefit from exercises that involve circular motions and lateral stretches. Hip joints, integral to mobility, thrive on stretches that encompass forward and lateral movements. The spine, a flexible yet stabilizing structure, benefits from exercises that promote both flexion and extension.

By incorporating joint-specific stretching into the routine, seniors cultivate a heightened awareness of each joint's capabilities and limitations. This approach not only enhances flexibility but also contributes to joint health and longevity.

Progressive Loading
Embracing a comprehensive range of motion involves a progressive loading strategy. Rather than static and abrupt movements, stretching exercises should gradually progress in intensity. This progression allows muscles and connective tissues to adapt and become more pliable over time.

Seniors are encouraged to start with gentle stretches and progressively increase the intensity as the body becomes accustomed. This might involve holding a stretch for a longer duration, increasing the range of motion, or incorporating resistance through props or bodyweight. The gradual nature of progressive loading minimizes the risk of injury while promoting a steady improvement in flexibility.

Functional Flexibility
The true essence of a comprehensive range of motion lies in functional flexibility. It's not just about reaching a certain degree of flexibility during a stretch; it's about applying that flexibility to real-life movements and activities. For seniors, functional flexibility directly translates to improved ease of performing daily tasks and maintaining an active lifestyle.

Functional flexibility exercises mimic the motions commonly encountered in daily life. This might include reaching for objects on shelves, bending to tie shoelaces, or twisting to look over the shoulder. By aligning stretching exercises with functional movements, seniors equip themselves with the flexibility needed to navigate the demands of daily living effortlessly.

Breathing Techniques for Enhanced Stretching

Breath, the life force that animates the body, becomes a powerful ally in the realm of stretching exercises. Intentional and mindful breathing techniques elevate the stretching experience from a physical routine to a holistic practice that engages both body and mind.

Diaphragmatic Breathing
At the core of breathing techniques for enhanced stretching is diaphragmatic breathing, often referred to as belly breathing. This technique involves engaging the diaphragm, the primary muscle responsible for breathing, to facilitate deep and controlled inhalation and exhalation.

Seniors are guided to initiate breaths from the diaphragm, allowing the abdomen to expand on inhalation and contract on exhalation. This intentional engagement of the diaphragm serves multiple purposes during stretching exercises. It promotes oxygenation of muscles, enhancing their performance and reducing the risk of cramping. Additionally, diaphragmatic breathing induces a sense of calm, fostering relaxation and mindfulness during stretching.

Synchronized Breathing

Incorporating synchronized breathing with movement amplifies the benefits of stretching exercises. This involves coordinating breath cycles with specific phases of a stretch. For example, inhaling during the initial phase of a stretch and exhaling during the release.

Synchronized breathing enhances the fluidity of movements, creating a seamless dance between breath and stretch. It promotes a sense of rhythm and harmony, preventing the stretching routine from feeling disjointed or rigid. Seniors find that synchronized breathing not only enhances the physical aspects of stretching but also deepens the mind-body connection.

Breath Awareness and Mindfulness
Beyond the mechanical aspects of breathing, breath awareness and mindfulness become integral components of the stretching experience. Seniors are encouraged to cultivate an acute awareness of their breath, observing its rhythm and quality. This heightened awareness serves as an anchor, grounding individuals in the present moment and fostering a state of mindfulness.

Mindfulness during stretching exercises involves directing full attention to the sensations, movements, and breath. It dissolves distractions and creates a mental space where individuals can fully engage with their bodies. The marriage of breath awareness and mindfulness transforms stretching from a routine task to a meditative practice, offering mental clarity and relaxation.

Integrating Principles for True Strength

In weaving together the principles of a comprehensive range of motion and intentional breathing, seniors embark on a journey that transcends the physical realm. Each stretch becomes a symphony of movements, orchestrated with precision and mindfulness. The joint-specific approach ensures that every component of the body contributes harmoniously, fostering overall joint health and flexibility.

Progressive loading becomes the guiding force, leading individuals on a gradual path towards enhanced flexibility without compromising safety. Functional flexibility emerges as the practical application of stretching, enabling seniors to infuse their daily activities with newfound ease and grace.

Breathing techniques, with their transformative power, elevate the stretching routine to a holistic practice. Diaphragmatic breathing oxygenates muscles, synchronized breathing enhances fluidity, and mindfulness creates a mental sanctuary. Together, these principles form the pillars of true strength, unlocking not just physical flexibility but a profound connection between body, breath, and mind.

As we navigate through the subsequent chapters, armed with these principles, seniors are poised to embrace stretching exercises as more than a regimen—it becomes a journey of self-discovery, resilience, and the unlocking of true strength.

Chapter 5

Chair-based Stretching

In the dance of flexibility and comfort, the chair takes center stage. Chapter 5, "Chair-based Stretching," unfolds a tapestry of gentle exercises designed for seated comfort, tailored specifically for seniors over 50. In the embrace of a chair, individuals discover a realm of possibilities that transcend traditional notions of stretching. This chapter delves into the essence of chair-based stretching, offering a repertoire of exercises that honor the body's need for support while adapting to diverse mobility levels with grace and inclusivity.

Gentle Exercises for Seated Comfort

The chair, often a symbol of rest, transforms into a sanctuary of movement in the world of chair-based stretching. These gentle exercises unfold as a symphony of comfort, inviting seniors to explore the expanses of flexibility without leaving the reassuring embrace of their seat.

Neck Stretches

Commencing with the pinnacle of mobility, neck stretches offer a gentle entry into chair-based exercises. Seniors are encouraged to sit comfortably, their spine aligned with the chair. Slow, controlled movements tilt the head forward and backward, from side to side, and in gentle rotations. These movements release tension in the neck muscles, fostering a sense of relaxation.

As the neck is a conduit for nerve signals to the entire body, these stretches not only enhance flexibility but also alleviate stress and tension. Seniors find solace in the rhythmic motions, a gentle nod to the importance of caring for the often-overlooked muscles of the neck.

Shoulder Rolls and Stretches

The shoulders, stalwart guardians of mobility, take their turn in the chair-based symphony. Seated comfortably, seniors engage in circular shoulder rolls, guiding the shoulders through a full range of motion. This exercise not only loosens tightness but also enhances blood circulation to the shoulder muscles.

Accompanying shoulder rolls are gentle stretches. Raising the arms laterally, seniors feel the stretch along the sides of the torso and shoulders. These exercises foster flexibility in the shoulder joints and the surrounding muscles, alleviating discomfort caused by prolonged periods of sitting.

Seated Spinal Twists

The spine, a pillar of support and flexibility, becomes the focus of seated spinal twists. Seated squarely in the chair, seniors inhale deeply, lengthening the spine, and exhale as they twist gently to one side, using the chair's backrest for support. This movement engages the muscles along the spine and promotes a supple, agile torso.

Seated spinal twists are not only about physical flexibility but also about enhancing digestion and promoting a sense of revitalization. The gentle compression and release of abdominal organs during the twists stimulate the digestive system, offering additional health benefits beyond flexibility.

Leg and Knee Lifts

The lower extremities, often impacted by reduced mobility, find liberation in chair-based leg and knee lifts. Seated at the edge of the chair, seniors lift one knee towards the chest, holding briefly before lowering it back down. This exercise strengthens the hip flexors and quadriceps while enhancing flexibility in the hip joint.

For those with limited mobility, variations of leg lifts while seated can be explored. Extending the leg straight or performing gentle ankle circles accommodates different levels of flexibility. The focus is not on reaching extremes but on embracing the range of motion that feels comfortable and beneficial.

Ankle and Foot Exercises

Completing the ensemble of seated comfort are ankle and foot exercises. With feet firmly planted on the ground, seniors perform ankle circles, flexing and pointing the toes, and gently rolling the ankles. These exercises promote flexibility in the ankle joint and strengthen the muscles of the lower leg.

For those who may find it challenging to reach the ground, simple toe-tapping exercises provide a delightful alternative. The rhythmic tapping not only improves ankle flexibility but also serves as a subtle cardiovascular boost.

Adapting Stretching to Different Mobility Levels

In the inclusive realm of chair-based stretching, adaptability becomes the guiding principle. Each individual, with their unique mobility levels, is invited to partake in the symphony of movements. Adapting stretching exercises ensures that the benefits of flexibility are accessible to all, regardless of where they are on their mobility journey.

Customizable Intensity

One of the inherent beauties of chair-based stretching lies in its customizable intensity. Seniors have the flexibility to adjust the range of motion, the duration of stretches, and the number of repetitions based on their comfort and mobility levels. The chair serves not as a constraint but as a supportive ally, allowing individuals to tailor the exercises to their unique needs.

For those new to chair-based stretching or individuals with limited mobility, starting with smaller movements and gradually increasing intensity over time is a recommended approach. This gradual progression not only ensures safety but also instills confidence in the individual's ability to engage in stretching exercises comfortably.

Incorporating Props for Support
The inclusion of props further enhances the adaptability of chair-based stretching. Simple additions like resistance bands, soft cushions, or small weights can provide additional support and challenge. For instance, incorporating a resistance band into arm stretches adds gentle resistance, enhancing the engagement of arm muscles.

Props also contribute to maintaining proper alignment during stretches. Placing a cushion behind the lower back during seated twists provides lumbar support, making the exercise more comfortable for individuals with lower back concerns. The strategic use of props transforms chair-based stretching into a personalized and effective routine.

Gradual Progression and Consistency
Adapting stretching exercises to different mobility levels involves a commitment to gradual progression and consistency. Seniors are encouraged to embrace a mindset of continuous improvement rather than seeking rapid transformations. This approach aligns with the natural progression of the body and minimizes the risk of strain or discomfort.

Consistency becomes the cornerstone of adapting stretching to different mobility levels. Regular engagement in chair-based stretching, even with minimal movements initially, yields cumulative benefits over time. The body responds positively to consistent, gentle stretching, gradually increasing flexibility and comfort.

Chair-based Symphony of Flexibility

In the realm of chair-based stretching, the chair becomes an instrument of empowerment, inviting individuals to participate in a symphony of flexibility. Gentle exercises, tailored for seated comfort, unfold as movements that respect the body's need for support and adapt to diverse mobility levels.

As seniors explore the soothing cadence of neck stretches, the invigorating rhythm of shoulder rolls, and the harmonious flow of spinal twists, they discover that flexibility need not be an elusive pursuit. The chair becomes a vehicle for inclusivity, where adaptability is celebrated, and each participant, regardless of their mobility level, finds a place in the symphony of stretching.

In the subsequent chapters, the journey continues, with the lessons learned from chair-based stretching serving as a foundation for unlocking true strength. Seniors are empowered to carry the principles of adaptability, comfort, and inclusivity into their broader stretching routine, embracing a path that resonates with their unique needs and aspirations.

Chapter 6

Standing and Balance Exercises

The shift from the comfort of a chair to the steadiness of an upright position marks a pivotal chapter in the journey of stretching for seniors. Chapter 6, "Standing and Balance Exercises," unfolds as a tale of strength and stability. Here, the focus transcends mere flexibility, delving into the symbiotic relationship between stretching, balance, and the art of standing tall. Seniors over 50 embark on a journey to strengthen stability, embracing a series of exercises that not only fortify the body but also enhance flexibility in upright positions.

Strengthening Stability through Stretching

In the realm of standing and balance exercises, stability becomes the bedrock upon which flexibility thrives. The body, upright and engaged, is challenged to find equilibrium, creating a dynamic interplay between strength and suppleness.

Wall-supported Leg Stretches

Commencing the exploration of standing stability are wall-supported leg stretches. Seniors are guided to stand with their back against a wall, feet hip-width apart. With one leg extended forward, they lean gently into the wall, feeling a stretch along the back of the extended leg. This exercise not only enhances flexibility in the hamstrings but also challenges stability as the body maintains alignment against the wall.

As individuals progress, the height of the leg lift can be adjusted, providing opportunities for continuous challenge and improvement. The support of the wall ensures a controlled environment, allowing seniors to focus on both the stretch and maintaining a stable posture.

Heel-to-Toe Walks

Heel-to-toe walks bring an element of balance and coordination into the realm of standing exercises. Seniors are encouraged to take small steps, placing the heel of one foot directly in front of the toes of the other foot with each step. This deliberate movement engages the muscles of the lower limbs and challenges the body's ability to maintain balance.

As individuals become more accustomed to heel-to-toe walks, the pace can be increased, introducing an element of dynamic stability. This exercise not only enhances leg flexibility but also fosters a sense of control and steadiness in an upright position.

Tree Pose for Balance and Flexibility

The tree pose, a classic yoga-inspired stance, emerges as a cornerstone of standing stability and flexibility. Seniors stand tall, shifting their weight onto one leg, while the sole of the opposite foot rests against the inner thigh or calf of the standing leg. The arms can be extended overhead or positioned in a prayer-like gesture at the chest.

The tree pose demands not only balance but also a gentle stretch along the inner thigh and hip of the raised leg. As individuals find their balance, the pose becomes an elegant fusion of strength and flexibility. Over time, seniors can experiment with variations, adapting the height of the raised foot to their comfort and gradually increasing the duration of the pose.

Enhancing Flexibility in Upright Positions

The transition from sitting to standing brings with it a unique set of challenges and rewards. Chapter 6 unfolds as a canvas for enhancing flexibility in upright positions, where the body stands tall, resilient, and open to the expansive possibilities of movement.

Calf Stretches

Upright flexibility finds expression in targeted calf stretches. Seniors stand facing a wall, placing their hands on the wall for support. With one foot stepped forward and the other foot extended straight behind, individuals lean gently into the wall, feeling a stretch along the calf of the extended leg.

Calf stretches not only improve flexibility in the lower leg but also contribute to ankle mobility. As individuals become accustomed to the stretch, they can experiment with subtly adjusting the angle of the back foot to target different areas of the calf muscle.

Quadriceps Stretch with Support

Strengthening stability while enhancing flexibility in the quadriceps unfolds through a supportive stance. Seniors stand near a chair or counter, holding onto the support with one hand. Bending one knee, they bring the heel towards the buttocks, feeling a stretch along the front of the thigh.

This exercise not only targets the quadriceps but also challenges balance and stability. As individuals progress, they can explore variations, such as gently pushing the hips forward to intensify the stretch or trying the exercise without support for brief intervals.

Forward Bend for Spinal Flexibility

The journey of upright flexibility extends to forward bends that engage the spine and promote suppleness. Seniors stand with feet hip-width apart, gently hinge at the hips, and allow the upper body to lower towards the floor. The hands can rest on the thighs, shins, or the floor, depending on individual flexibility.

Forward bends contribute to spinal flexibility, elongating the muscles along the back and fostering a sense of decompression. The controlled descent and ascent in this exercise also enhance core strength, adding an extra layer to the interplay between stability and flexibility.

The Dance of Stability and Flexibility

In the choreography of standing and balance exercises, stability and flexibility perform a dance that celebrates the body's ability to stand tall and move with grace. Each stretch, each deliberate shift of weight, becomes a step in this dance, harmonizing the strength required to stand with the suppleness needed for graceful movement.

Mindful Alignment
Mindful alignment becomes a guiding principle in the realm of standing exercises. Seniors are encouraged to pay attention to the alignment of their spine, hips, and shoulders, ensuring that the body stands tall with integrity. Mindful alignment not only enhances the effectiveness of each stretch but also contributes to overall posture and body awareness.

Controlled Breathing for Focus
As the body engages in the dance of stability and flexibility, controlled breathing becomes a focal point. Seniors are guided to synchronize breath with movement, inhaling deeply during the initial phase of a stretch and exhaling as they return to the starting position. Controlled breathing enhances focus, creates a rhythm in movement, and fosters a sense of calm amidst the dynamic nature of standing exercises.

Standing Tall in True Strength

As Chapter 6 unfolds, seniors discover the transformative power of standing and balance exercises. The body, once confined to the support of a chair, rises to the occasion, standing tall and resilient. Stability and flexibility, once distant companions, find unity in the upright position, creating a holistic approach to true strength.

With the principles of strengthening stability through stretching and enhancing flexibility in upright positions, seniors over 50 cultivate a sense of empowerment. Each stretch becomes a brushstroke on the canvas of their journey, painting a portrait of resilience, balance, and the unwavering ability to stand tall in the pursuit of true strength.

As the narrative unfolds into subsequent chapters, the lessons learned from standing and balance exercises become threads woven into the fabric of the broader stretching routine. Seniors carry with them the dance of stability and flexibility, creating a tapestry of strength that extends beyond the physical realm—embracing a life of vitality, balance, and the unwavering capacity to stand tall in the face of time.

Chapter 7

Full-Body Stretching Routines

The culmination of the stretching journey for seniors unfolds in the expansive landscape of Chapter 7: Full-Body Stretching Routines. Here, the focus shifts to integrated approaches for comprehensive flexibility. The body, now familiar with chair-based stretches, standing exercises, and the dance of stability, takes center stage for a harmonious symphony of stretches that transcend individual muscle groups. This chapter becomes a canvas for building a personalized stretching routine, where each stretch seamlessly intertwines to create a tapestry of true strength.

Integrated Approaches for Comprehensive Flexibility

As seniors navigate the realm of full-body stretching, the emphasis shifts from isolated movements to integrated approaches that engage multiple muscle groups simultaneously. Comprehensive flexibility becomes the goal, weaving together the threads of various stretches into a cohesive, transformative experience.

Dynamic Warm-up Sequences

Embarking on a full-body stretching routine necessitates an orchestrated warm-up that prepares the body for the symphony of stretches to come. Dynamic warm-up sequences serve as the overture, gently awakening muscles, increasing blood flow, and priming joints for the forthcoming movements.

Seniors engage in dynamic movements that mimic the actions of the stretching routine. This might include arm circles, leg swings, torso twists, and gentle marching in place. The dynamic nature of these warm-up sequences not only readies the body physically but also serves as a transition into a focused, mindful state—a precursor to the holistic experience of full-body stretching.

Neck-to-Toe Flexibility Flow
The centerpiece of full-body stretching unfolds as a neck-to-toe flexibility flow—a sequence that transcends the traditional compartmentalization of stretches. Seniors begin by gently tilting the head forward, allowing the stretch to cascade down the spine. With each movement, the focus shifts progressively from one area of the body to the next, creating a fluid dance of flexibility.

The neck-to-toe flexibility flow includes stretches for the neck, shoulders, spine, hips, legs, and ankles, seamlessly transitioning from one to the next. This integrated approach ensures that every part of the body participates in the dynamic stretch, fostering a sense of interconnectedness and balance.

Flowing Yoga-inspired Poses
Yoga, with its centuries-old wisdom, becomes a source of inspiration for full-body stretching routines. Flowing through yoga-inspired poses adds a layer of mindfulness and intentional movement to the routine. Seniors engage in poses such as Downward-Facing Dog, Warrior I, and Cat-Cow, allowing the body to explore diverse ranges of motion and stretch multiple muscle groups simultaneously.

Yoga-inspired poses not only contribute to flexibility but also enhance balance and stability. The deliberate transitions between poses encourage a mind-body connection, fostering a sense of presence and awareness. As seniors gracefully flow through these poses, they embody the essence of full-body flexibility—a journey that transcends the physical and touches the realms of mindfulness.

Building a Personalized Stretching Routine

In the tapestry of full-body stretching, personalization becomes the brushstroke that adds uniqueness to the journey. Building a personalized stretching routine is an art—a reflection of individual preferences, challenges, and aspirations.

Assessing Individual Needs
The foundation of a personalized stretching routine lies in assessing individual needs. Seniors are encouraged to reflect on their bodies, considering areas of stiffness, past injuries, and specific goals. This introspective assessment forms the blueprint for tailoring the routine to address personal requirements and aspirations.

For example, someone with a history of lower back discomfort may choose to incorporate additional stretches for the lower back and hips. Alternatively, an individual seeking improved posture might prioritize stretches that engage the muscles of the upper back and shoulders. The personalized routine becomes a compass, guiding individuals towards stretches that align with their unique journey.

Embracing Variability
Flexibility is not a static state but a dynamic quality that evolves over time. Embracing variability becomes a key principle in building a personalized stretching routine. Seniors are encouraged to experiment with different stretches, vary the duration and intensity, and explore a diverse range of movements.

Variability not only prevents monotony but also promotes a well-rounded approach to flexibility. Incorporating stretches that target different planes of movement and muscle groups ensures comprehensive coverage, contributing to overall flexibility and joint health.

Setting Realistic Goals

In the realm of personalized stretching, setting realistic and achievable goals provides a sense of purpose and direction. Seniors are guided to identify specific areas for improvement, whether it be increased range of motion in a particular joint, enhanced flexibility in a muscle group, or addressing posture-related concerns.

Realistic goals serve as beacons, guiding the frequency and intensity of the stretching routine. As individuals witness incremental progress towards these goals, they experience a sense of accomplishment and motivation, fueling their commitment to the ongoing journey of flexibility.

Tailoring Frequency and Duration

The frequency and duration of the stretching routine are personal choices that align with individual preferences and schedules. Seniors are empowered to tailor these aspects to suit their lifestyle, recognizing that consistency is key to reaping the benefits of flexibility.

For some, a daily brief stretching routine may be feasible, while others may prefer longer sessions a few times a week. The key is to strike a balance that is sustainable and enjoyable. The routine should be a source of rejuvenation rather than a chore, fostering a positive relationship with the practice of flexibility.

The Tapestry of True Strength

As Chapter 7 unfolds, the full-body stretching routine emerges as a tapestry—a carefully woven composition of integrated approaches, personalization, and the unwavering commitment to true strength. Seniors, now well-versed in the art of stretching, find themselves standing at the intersection of flexibility and mindfulness.

Mindful Presence

Full-body stretching becomes a gateway to mindful presence—a state where individuals are fully engaged in the present moment. Each stretch becomes a conscious movement, each breath an anchor that ties the mind to the body. Mindful presence transcends the physicality of stretching, creating an opportunity for introspection and self-awareness.

Resilience and Adaptability

In the journey of building a personalized stretching routine, seniors cultivate resilience and adaptability. The routine becomes a testament to the body's capacity to adapt, evolve, and embrace change. As individuals navigate through different stretches, experiment with variability, and set and achieve realistic goals, they embody the qualities of resilience and adaptability that extend beyond the realm of flexibility.

The Unveiling of True Strength

The tapestry of full-body stretching routines becomes the unveiling of true strength—a strength that extends beyond the physical to encompass mental fortitude, emotional well-being, and a profound connection with one's body. Seniors discover that true strength is not a destination but a continuous journey—one that unfolds with each intentional stretch, each personalized routine, and each moment of mindful presence.

As the narrative concludes, seniors carry with them the lessons learned from full-body stretching, weaving these insights into the fabric of their daily lives. The tapestry of true strength becomes a living testament to the transformative power of flexibility—a power that enhances not only the body but also the spirit, creating a harmonious symphony that resonates with vitality, resilience, and the unwavering commitment to unlock true strength.

Chapter 8

Targeted Stretches for Common Concerns

In the tapestry of stretching for seniors, Chapter 8 unfolds as a tailored guide—offering targeted stretches for common concerns that often accompany the golden years. Alleviating joint stiffness and enhancing posture and mobility become the central themes, providing a roadmap for seniors over 50 to address specific challenges with precision and care. This chapter delves into the intricacies of targeted stretches, empowering individuals to unlock their true strength by addressing common concerns that may arise on their journey to flexibility.

Alleviating Joint Stiffness

As time unfolds, joints may bear the weight of accumulated experiences, leading to stiffness and reduced mobility. Chapter 8 becomes a sanctuary for those seeking relief—a collection of targeted stretches designed to alleviate joint stiffness and restore a sense of fluidity and ease.

Neck and Shoulder Release

The neck and shoulders, often harboring tension and stiffness, find solace in a series of targeted stretches. Seniors are guided through gentle neck tilts, side stretches, and shoulder rolls, allowing the muscles around the neck and shoulders to unwind. These stretches not only alleviate stiffness but also promote relaxation, creating a serene haven for individuals carrying the burdens of the day.

For those with specific concerns such as tightness in the trapezius or neck discomfort, targeted stretches like the chin tuck—a subtle movement that involves gently bringing the chin towards the chest—provide a focused release. These stretches can be tailored to address individual areas of tension, offering a personalized approach to alleviating joint stiffness.

Wrist and Hand Flexibility
The hands and wrists, vital in daily activities, may encounter stiffness, especially for those engaged in repetitive motions. Targeted stretches for wrist and hand flexibility become essential in promoting comfort and preserving dexterity.

Seniors engage in exercises that involve gentle wrist circles, finger stretches, and palm presses. These stretches enhance flexibility in the hands and wrists, alleviating stiffness that may arise from prolonged periods of typing, writing, or engaging in manual tasks. The incorporation of these targeted stretches contributes not only to joint health but also to the overall functionality of the hands.

Hip Opener Stretches
The hips, pivotal in maintaining balance and mobility, can often be a source of stiffness, particularly for those with sedentary lifestyles. Targeted hip opener stretches offer a gateway to increased flexibility and reduced discomfort.

Seniors partake in exercises such as seated hip stretches, hip circles, and knee-to-chest stretches. These movements gently open up the hips, encouraging a greater range of motion. For those experiencing specific hip concerns, modifications and variations cater to individual needs, ensuring that the stretches are both accessible and effective in alleviating joint stiffness.

Improving Posture and Mobility

Posture, a silent ally in the journey of aging gracefully, becomes a focal point in Chapter 8. Targeted stretches for improving posture and mobility not only address physical concerns but also contribute to a sense of poise, confidence, and overall well-being.

Chest Opener Stretches
A forward-leaning posture, often exacerbated by prolonged periods of sitting, can lead to rounded shoulders and a compressed chest. Targeted chest opener stretches offer a remedy, creating space in the chest and promoting an upright posture.

Seniors engage in exercises that involve gentle backbends, shoulder blade squeezes, and wall stretches. These movements expand the chest, counteracting the effects of slouching and promoting improved posture. The targeted nature of these stretches allows individuals to focus on the specific areas that contribute to postural concerns, fostering a sense of openness and alignment.

Thoracic Spine Mobility
The thoracic spine, situated in the upper and mid-back, plays a crucial role in maintaining mobility and preventing stiffness. Targeted stretches for thoracic spine mobility become a cornerstone in improving overall posture and addressing concerns related to upper back discomfort.

Seniors partake in exercises such as seated twists, cat-cow stretches, and thoracic extensions. These stretches focus on creating gentle movement in the upper back, fostering flexibility and relieving tension. For those with specific concerns such as stiffness between the shoulder blades, variations in these stretches provide an opportunity for targeted relief.

Lower Back and Hip Flexor Stretches
The lower back and hip flexors bear the brunt of sedentary lifestyles and may contribute to issues such as lower back pain and compromised mobility. Targeted stretches for the lower back and hip flexors become essential in promoting flexibility and alleviating discomfort.

Seniors engage in exercises that involve gentle forward bends, seated hip flexor stretches, and figure-four stretches. These movements target the muscles around the lower back and hips, encouraging suppleness and reducing tension. The targeted nature of these stretches provides individuals with the tools to address specific concerns related to lower back and hip discomfort.

Tailoring Targeted Stretches to Individual Needs

In the realm of targeted stretches for common concerns, personalization is key. Chapter 8 encourages seniors to tailor these stretches to their individual needs, recognizing that each body is unique and requires a bespoke approach to flexibility.

Assessing Specific Concerns
The first step in tailoring targeted stretches involves a thoughtful assessment of specific concerns. Seniors are guided to identify areas of stiffness, discomfort, or challenges related to posture and mobility. This self-awareness forms the foundation for selecting stretches that directly address individual needs.

For example, someone experiencing persistent wrist discomfort may prioritize wrist and hand flexibility stretches, while another individual with concerns about rounded shoulders might focus on chest opener stretches. The process of assessment allows seniors to approach flexibility with intention, creating a targeted routine that aligns with their unique journey.

Incorporating Modifications and Props

Personalization extends to incorporating modifications and props that enhance the effectiveness of targeted stretches. Seniors are encouraged to explore variations of stretches, adjusting the intensity, duration, or positioning based on their comfort and ability.

For instance, using a cushion or rolled towel under the wrists during hand and wrist stretches can provide additional support and comfort. Similarly, incorporating a chair or wall for stability during hip opener stretches ensures a safe and accessible practice. The inclusion of modifications and props transforms targeted stretches into a customizable and adaptable routine.

Gradual Progression and Consistency

Tailoring targeted stretches involves a commitment to gradual progression and consistency. Seniors are reminded that flexibility is a journey, and the goal is not to achieve rapid transformations but to experience sustainable and long-lasting benefits.

Individuals are encouraged to start with stretches that match their current level of flexibility and gradually progress over time. Consistent engagement in targeted stretches, even with smaller movements initially, yields cumulative benefits, fostering improved posture, reduced stiffness, and enhanced mobility.

The Transformation of Concerns into Strength

As Chapter 8 reaches its crescendo, targeted stretches for common concerns become a transformative tool—a means to turn areas of discomfort into reservoirs of strength. Seniors, armed with a personalized understanding of their bodies and a repertoire of stretches tailored to their needs, embark on a journey of alleviating joint stiffness, improving posture, and enhancing overall mobility.

Empowerment Through Awareness

The process of tailoring targeted stretches empowers seniors through awareness—a heightened understanding of their bodies, concerns, and the potential for positive change. Awareness becomes a beacon that guides individuals towards stretches that offer targeted relief and contribute to the overarching goal of unlocking true strength.

A Holistic Approach to Flexibility

The targeted stretches presented in Chapter 8 contribute to a holistic approach to flexibility—one that addresses specific concerns while recognizing the interconnectedness of the body. The neck, shoulders, wrists, hips, and spine are not isolated entities but integral components of a dynamic whole. Targeted stretches serve as threads woven into the intricate fabric of overall flexibility.

The Ripple Effect of True Strength

As seniors experience the benefits of targeted stretches, a ripple effect of true strength permeates their lives. Alleviated joint stiffness allows for a greater range of motion, improved posture instills confidence, and enhanced mobility fosters a sense of freedom. The targeted stretches become catalysts for a life marked by vitality, resilience, and the unwavering commitment to unlocking true strength.

In the subsequent chapters, seniors continue their journey, armed with the knowledge and practice of targeted stretches. The lessons learned become an enduring guide, shaping a path of flexibility that aligns with individual needs, aspirations, and the ever-evolving tapestry of true strength.

Chapter 9

Incorporating Stretching into Daily Life

As the journey through the essential guide to stretching for seniors unfolds, Chapter 9 emerges as a compass guiding individuals to seamlessly weave stretching into the fabric of their daily lives. The focus sharpens on making stretching not just a routine but a habit—a harmonious integration into the rhythm of each day. This chapter becomes a testament to the transformative power of consistency, illustrating how the simple act of making stretching a daily habit can unlock true strength and foster a life of enduring flexibility.

The Essence of Daily Integration

Incorporating stretching into daily life is more than a series of isolated exercises—it is a conscious choice to infuse moments of flexibility into the very fabric of each day. Chapter 9 explores the essence of daily integration, inviting seniors to embrace a lifestyle where stretching becomes as natural as breathing.

Morning Awakening Routine
The morning, with its promise of a new day, becomes an opportune canvas for stretching. A morning awakening routine, carefully designed to gently invigorate the body, sets the tone for a day filled with vitality and flexibility.

Seniors engage in a sequence of stretches that cater to the body's awakening state—gentle neck stretches, shoulder rolls, and ankle circles. The goal is not to perform elaborate movements but to create a mindful transition from sleep to wakefulness. Incorporating stretches that target major muscle groups promotes blood circulation, reduces stiffness, and provides an energizing start to the day.

Stretch Breaks Throughout the Day
Amidst the demands of daily life, stretch breaks become anchors—moments of reprieve that infuse flexibility into routine tasks. Chapter 9 encourages seniors to incorporate short stretch breaks throughout the day, whether at the desk, in the kitchen, or during moments of leisure.

For those spending extended periods at a desk, simple seated stretches, neck rotations, and wrist flexor stretches offer relief from the sedentary posture. In the kitchen, waiting for the kettle to boil becomes an opportunity for calf raises or gentle leg stretches. These micro-stretch breaks not only contribute to overall flexibility but also serve as mindful pauses that rejuvenate both body and mind.

Evening Unwinding Ritual
As the day gracefully winds down, an evening unwinding ritual emerges—a sanctuary of stretching that prepares the body for restful sleep. The stretches in this sequence are designed to release tension accumulated throughout the day and promote a sense of relaxation.

Seniors engage in calming stretches such as gentle forward bends, seated twists, and slow, deliberate breathing exercises. The emphasis shifts from invigorating movements to soothing stretches that encourage a mind-body connection. The evening unwinding ritual becomes a bridge between the active moments of the day and the restorative serenity of the night.

Making Stretching a Habit

The transformation of stretching from a sporadic practice to a daily habit requires intention, commitment, and an understanding of the psychological and physiological aspects of habit formation. Chapter 9 delves into the art of making stretching a habit, exploring strategies that transcend mere routine and become ingrained in the fabric of daily life.

Setting Clear Intentions

The journey towards making stretching a habit begins with setting clear intentions. Seniors are encouraged to articulate why stretching is important to them—whether it be for improved flexibility, reduced discomfort, or enhanced overall well-being.

Clear intentions serve as the foundation for the habit-building process, creating a sense of purpose and motivation. Individuals are invited to reflect on how the benefits of stretching align with their personal goals and aspirations. This clarity becomes a compass, guiding them through the initial phases of habit formation.

Start Small and Gradual Progression

In the quest to make stretching a daily habit, the principle of starting small takes center stage. Seniors are guided to initiate the habit with a manageable and realistic commitment—perhaps a brief morning routine or a couple of stretch breaks during the day.

Starting small ensures that the habit is approachable and minimizes the potential for overwhelm. Once the initial habit is established, gradual progression becomes the next step. Individuals can incrementally add more stretches, increase the duration, or explore different routines as they become more accustomed to incorporating stretching into their daily lives.

Anchor to Existing Habits

Anchoring stretching to existing habits serves as a powerful strategy for habit formation. Seniors are encouraged to identify routine activities or cues in their daily lives and attach stretching to these anchors.

For example, stretching could become a ritual after morning coffee, a break between work tasks, or before bedtime. The association with existing habits helps integrate stretching seamlessly, transforming it from a standalone activity to an integral part of daily routines. Anchoring to existing habits leverages the familiarity of established routines, facilitating the assimilation of stretching into the rhythm of daily life.

Create a Dedicated Space

Designating a specific space for stretching contributes to the establishment of a habit. Whether it's a corner in the living room, a quiet spot in the bedroom, or a comfortable chair for chair-based stretches, having a dedicated space creates a visual and physical cue for the habit of stretching.

Seniors are encouraged to personalize this space with elements that evoke a sense of tranquility and motivation. It could be a favorite stretching mat, soothing music, or natural light streaming through a window. The act of creating a dedicated space elevates the significance of stretching, reinforcing its place in daily life.

The Psychology of Habit Formation

Understanding the psychology of habit formation becomes instrumental in making stretching a seamless part of daily life. Chapter 9 explores the underlying principles that govern habit formation, shedding light on the cognitive and behavioral aspects that contribute to the sustainability of the stretching habit.

Consistency and the Habit Loop

The habit loop, consisting of cue, routine, and reward, serves as a blueprint for understanding and cultivating habits. Seniors are guided to identify a cue—a trigger that initiates the stretching routine. This could be a specific time of day, an environmental cue, or an emotional state.

The routine, in this case, is the stretching itself—a series of intentional movements designed to enhance flexibility. The reward is the positive feeling that follows the stretching routine—whether it's a sense of rejuvenation, reduced discomfort, or the satisfaction of completing a beneficial activity.

Consistency is the linchpin that reinforces the habit loop. The more consistently individuals engage in the stretching routine, the stronger the habit becomes. As the habit loop becomes ingrained in daily life, stretching transforms from a deliberate practice to an automatic response, seamlessly integrated into the rhythm of each day.

Positive Reinforcement

Positive reinforcement plays a pivotal role in habit formation. Seniors are encouraged to celebrate small victories and acknowledge the positive impact of stretching on their well-being. Positive reinforcement creates an association between the stretching habit and feelings of accomplishment and satisfaction.

This could involve keeping a stretching journal to track progress, setting milestone rewards for consistent stretching, or simply acknowledging the moments of joy and rejuvenation that accompany the habit. The act of recognizing and celebrating the positive aspects of stretching reinforces the habit, making it more likely to endure.

Overcoming Challenges with Mindful Resilience
In the journey of making stretching a habit, challenges may arise—whether they be time constraints, fluctuations in motivation, or unforeseen disruptions to routines. Chapter 9 introduces the concept of mindful resilience—a mindset that acknowledges challenges without succumbing to defeat.

Seniors are guided to approach challenges with curiosity and a non-judgmental attitude. Instead of viewing a missed stretching session as a failure, they are encouraged to explore the underlying reasons and adapt the habit to changing circumstances. Mindful resilience fosters a flexible and adaptable approach to habit formation, allowing individuals to navigate challenges with grace and perseverance.

The Tapestry of Daily Integration

As Chapter 9 reaches its culmination, the integration of stretching into daily life becomes a living tapestry—a mosaic of intentional choices, habits, and the unwavering commitment to unlock true strength. Seniors, now adept at seamlessly incorporating stretching into their daily routines, stand at the intersection of routine and transformation.

A Lifestyle of Flexibility
In making stretching a habit, seniors cultivate a lifestyle of flexibility that extends beyond the physical realm. The habitual integration of stretching becomes a reflection of a mindset—a commitment to prioritize self-care, well-being, and the enduring pursuit of true strength.

Mindful Presence in Daily Rituals

The tapestry of daily integration is woven with threads of mindful presence. Seniors discover that each stretch, each moment of intentional movement, becomes an opportunity for mindfulness—a presence that transcends the habitual and connects them to the richness of each day.

A Lifetime of True Strength

As individuals continue to navigate the tapestry of daily integration, the habit of stretching becomes a companion for a lifetime. The journey extends beyond the pages of Chapter 9, permeating the years to come with the enduring essence of true strength.

In the subsequent chapters, seniors carry with them the art and wisdom of daily integration. The lessons learned become an enduring guide, shaping a path of flexibility that aligns with the ever-evolving tapestry of true strength—a tapestry that is not only witnessed but actively woven, thread by intentional thread, in the fabric of a life well-lived.

Conclusion

Unlocking Your True Strength

As the final chapter unfolds, it marks not just the conclusion of a comprehensive guide but the commencement of a transformative journey for seniors over 50— a journey to unlock true strength through the essential guide to stretching for enhanced flexibility. The pages have been woven with insights, exercises, and wisdom, creating a tapestry that transcends the physical and reaches into the realms of resilience, mindfulness, and enduring well-being.

Reflection on the Journey

The journey embarked upon in this guide is more than a series of stretching exercises; it is a holistic exploration of what it means to age with vitality, grace, and a commitment to self-care. Seniors have traversed the landscape of stretching, discovering not just the mechanics of flexibility but the profound interconnectedness of mind, body, and spirit.

Reflecting on the journey, it's evident that unlocking true strength is not a destination but a continuous, intentional process. Each stretch, each routine, and each moment of mindful presence contribute to a life richly lived. Seniors have become artists of their own well-being, painting strokes of resilience, balance, and the unwavering capacity to stand tall in the face of time.

Embracing the Benefits of Stretching

The guide commenced with an exploration of the benefits of stretching, inviting seniors to embrace the transformative power of intentional movement. From improved flexibility and joint health to enhanced posture and mental well-being, each stretch became a gateway to a life of vitality. Seniors have experienced the tangible benefits of stretching, witnessing the positive impact on their bodies, minds, and overall quality of life.

Understanding Senior Fitness

Chapter by chapter, the guide delved into the nuances of senior fitness, addressing the changes in flexibility that accompany the graceful process of aging. Understanding senior fitness became a key pillar, empowering individuals to approach stretching with awareness and tailored consideration for their unique needs. Aging gracefully, as explored in Chapter 2, became a journey marked by adaptability, acceptance, and the unwavering commitment to prioritize one's well-being.

Getting Started Safely

The guide provided a solid foundation in Chapter 3, ensuring seniors could embark on their stretching journey safely and with confidence. Preparing for stretching and incorporating warm-up techniques became integral steps, fostering a mindful approach to movement. Seniors learned to listen to their bodies, pacing themselves and cultivating a relationship with stretching that prioritizes safety and well-being.

Key Stretching Principles

Chapter 4 unveiled the key stretching principles that underpin a comprehensive approach to flexibility. Seniors explored the nuances of range of motion and discovered the transformative potential of breathing techniques. These principles became guiding lights, illuminating the path towards a well-rounded stretching routine that embraces the subtleties of intentional movement.

Chair-based Stretching

In Chapter 5, the guide introduced chair-based stretching, recognizing the diversity of mobility levels among seniors. Gentle exercises for seated comfort became a bridge, ensuring that stretching remains accessible to individuals with varying physical abilities. Seniors explored adaptability, learning that the essence of stretching lies not in the complexity of the movement but in the intention behind each stretch.

Standing and Balance Exercises

Chapter 6 elevated the journey with standing and balance exercises, introducing the dynamic interplay between stability and flexibility. Seniors engaged in movements that strengthened stability while enhancing flexibility in upright positions. Each exercise became a brushstroke on the canvas of their journey, painting a portrait of resilience, balance, and the unwavering ability to stand tall in the pursuit of true strength.

Full-Body Stretching Routines

The culmination of the stretching journey unfolded in Chapter 7, where integrated approaches for comprehensive flexibility took center stage. Seniors explored dynamic warm-up sequences, neck-to-toe flexibility flows, and flowing yoga-inspired poses. The chapter became a canvas for building personalized full-body stretching routines, where each stretch seamlessly intertwined into a tapestry of true strength.

Targeted Stretches for Common Concerns

Chapter 8 provided a tailored guide, offering targeted stretches for common concerns that accompany the golden years. Seniors discovered the art of alleviating joint stiffness and improving posture and mobility through a series of intentional stretches. The chapter became a transformative tool, allowing areas of discomfort to be turned into reservoirs of strength through personalized flexibility.

Incorporating Stretching into Daily Life

The guide reached the zenith of practical wisdom in Chapter 9, where stretching transformed from a routine to a habit seamlessly woven into daily life. Seniors explored the essence of daily integration, making stretching a part of morning awakenings, stretch breaks throughout the day, and evening unwinding rituals. Making stretching a habit became an art, an intentional choice that echoed in the rhythm of each day.

The Journey Continues

As the guide concludes, it marks not the end but a transition—an invitation for seniors to carry the lessons learned into the fabric of their lives. The journey continues beyond the pages, with each stretch contributing to a lifetime of true strength. Seniors are empowered with the tools, knowledge, and mindset to navigate the ever-evolving tapestry of flexibility with grace, resilience, and a commitment to unlocking their true strength.

The Unveiling of True Strength

In the tapestry of stretching for seniors over 50, true strength is unveiled—not as a singular achievement but as a continuous journey. It is a journey marked by flexibility, resilience, and a commitment to well-being. Seniors stand at the intersection of the physical and the mindful, embodying the essence of true strength—a strength that extends beyond the body to encompass the spirit.

A Gratitude for the Stretching Journey

As the final words unfold, there's a profound gratitude for the stretching journey embarked upon together. Seniors are invited to carry the wisdom gained, the habits formed, and the resilience cultivated into the chapters that lie ahead. The guide concludes, not as a farewell, but as a celebration of the enduring pursuit of true strength—a pursuit that echoes in the stretches, routines, and mindful moments that weave into the fabric of a life enriched by flexibility.

Thanks for reading this book and don't hesitate to give me a review about the book